Modern Bodybuilding and Fat Loss Techniques

The DACT Method to Success

Nicholas Kondisenko B.Bus(Hons) & B.IT

2015

First Edition.
Designed by Nicholas Kondisenko.

ISBN-13: 978-1481213707
ISBN-10: 1481213709

You are about to embark on one of the most exciting personal adventures of your life. You will transform your body into a more muscular, toned and lean physique. You will be healthier, fitter and more flexible. The DACT method has transformed the lives of teenagers to retirees. You will be stronger and have the ability to overcome any obstacle that presents itself in your life. Because you will be fit and strong, you'll overcome these obstacles that you once thought were impossible. All you have to do is put the DACT method to work for you, stick to your training and nutrition, focus on your goals and achieve the body that you so much deserve.

Nicholas Kondisenko.

Contents

Acknowledgements

This book is not the end of my journey; it is just the beginning…for you and me, it is a journey of self-fulfillment, continual learning and bettering oneself to reach the highest echelons which we thought were impossible.

It is an opportunity for me to share the knowledge and experience of over 20 years' worth of Bodybuilding and fitness and to express my personal flair on these pages.

First and foremost, to my wife Oli and my two beautiful children Rhiannon and Alex, without you my life would be empty. You have given me unconditional support in everything that I do, whether it is bodybuilding, music, painting, study or just hanging out to watch a movie. I am so proud to be your husband and father and try to be the best role model that I can be. You can be and do anything in this life, just have a go. I love you with all my heart.

To my parents, for your love and support throughout my life. You had your doubts, but you stuck by me and it all come good in the end.

To my Nonno Peter, I miss you.

How it all Began

Thinking back, I guess the first encounter with Bodybuilding or the act of lifting weights began when I was about ten. I recall one weekend, while I was kicking around the yard, a distinctively loud bang from my next door neighbors shed. Being an inquisitive young lad, I quickly jumped the fence to see what was going on. To my amazement, my young neighbor John had dropped a heavily loaded barbell onto the side of his parent's car and left a huge dent in the left hand front fender. He had this homemade weight set of what seemed at the time, massive lumps of steel which he had fashioned while working as an apprentice at the sugar mill.

I had asked him what he was doing and he explained to me about lifting weights and bodybuilding. He then asked me "do you want to workout?" and I quickly replied "cool" as only a ten year old could. After a few weeks I had begun to notice my muscles were getting bigger, especially my legs. My lower quads were becoming quite muscular. I have to admit though my legs were always my strong point.

Throughout my high school years I was always actively involved in sports and martial arts, specifically Kung Fu. I progressed to Light Blue belt and found that I needed more strength. So my good mate Ian introduced me to the Gym. It was 1987 that I officially can call my starting point as a bodybuilder at Gold's Gym Townsville. From that moment on I was hooked.

The Classic Era
Bodybuilding (the art of displaying the muscles) did not really exist prior to the late 19th century, when it was promoted by a man from Prussia named Eugen Sandow,

who is now generally referred to as "The Father of Modern Bodybuilding".(Gwillim, 2012)

Eugen Sandow changed the way we see and think about our bodies. Although he was born a century and a half ago, his actions still live with us today. He made physical fitness palatable to the multitudes, inspiring countless others to become athletes themselves. Sandow burst upon the athletic scene with all the force and brilliance of a shooting star, blazing as if from nowhere into the Victorian sporting and theatrical world. He became the great teacher, and performer who helped transform bodybuilding from the occupation of a few faithful devotees to the esteemed sport that it is today.

Before Sandow started his strongman act on the London stage, most people thought that a muscleman had to look like a cross between John Candy and King Kong. Sandow showed the world that he could be strong and at the same time muscled and well proportioned. This blond, blue-eyed athlete became a matinee idol decades before Steve Reeves or Arnold Schwarzenegger. Young ladies would flock around the vestibule counter wherever he performed, eager to buy photographs of his scantily clad image. Even the men seemed to have been caught up in the general enthusiasm over this striking young strongman. "He is positively handsome in form, feature, face, and limb," one journalist crowed. "He is the beau-ideal of athletic elegance." But we must also remember that Sandow was more than just another pretty face...much more.(Chapman, 2012)

Classic bodybuilding evokes a variety of mental images, from 19th century muscle men in striped trunks to Arnold Schwarzenegger pumping iron in the 1970s. This unofficial classic era, which lasted nearly a century, differed greatly from the modern form of bodybuilding that has exploded since the 1980s. Factors, such as science and commercialization, have helped turn bodybuilding from a fringe novelty into a multi-billion dollar, worldwide industry.(Howells, 2012)

Modern Bodybuilding
One of the biggest differences between modern and classic bodybuilding, and perhaps the key distinguishing feature between the two eras, relates to aesthetics. Old photographs of bodybuilders from around the turn of the 20th century reveal large and clearly strong men, but not the kind of muscle definition that is so characteristic of the modern athlete. Organized competition and international organizations have promoted more rigid definitions of what successful bodybuilding should look like, and this unified goal has been the catalyst for many of the other developments made in the sport.(Howells, 2012)

When we think of modern bodybuilding the majority of people will claim Arnold Schwarzenegger and the movie Pumping Iron to be the start. To the average person, Arnold was the panicle of modern physiques; bought to the masses by the big movie screen and great movies such as Commando, Predator, and the Terminator series. But in all reality, if it wasn't for siblings Ben and Joe Weider, bodybuilding would not exist as it is today.

Josef E. "Joe" Weider (born November 29, 1919) is co-founder of the International Federation of Bodybuilders (IFBB) along with brother Ben Weider and creator of the Mr. Olympia, the Ms. Olympia, and the now-defunct Masters Olympia bodybuilding contests. He is the publisher of several bodybuilding and fitness-related magazines, most notably Muscle and Fitness, Flex, Men's Fitness and

Shape, and is the manufacturer of a line of fitness equipment and fitness supplements.(Wikipedia, 2012b)

From a small, shabby warehouse in Brooklyn, New York, Joe established a magazine empire. By 1952, 'Your Physique' reached record sales levels and prompted Weider to distribute 20 separate magazines with a total circulation of about 25 million readers. (Hoxha, 1995)

'Your Physique', which he renamed 'Muscle Builder' reached a respectable 80,000 monthly circulation by 1965, allowing the Weiders to focus their energies on bolstering the sport of bodybuilding. The sport was losing many of its top competitors, who were forced to take jobs as bouncers, bodyguards and professional wrestlers because they couldn't make a living in the sport of their choice. By increasing contest incomes, the Weiders' hoped to keep both veterans and rising champions in the sport.(Hoxha, 1995)

They subsequently created the Mr. Olympia contest to showcase bodybuilder's top talent in the hope of attracting lucrative television and business contracts that would support the fledgling sport. Yet the deals didn't materialize. In the mid-'60s, advertisers still considered bodybuilding a cult sport practiced by 'muscleheads', and having little mainstream appeal.(Hoxha, 1995)

The National Physique Committee (NPC) was formed in 1981 by Jim Manion,(Jim Manion, 2007-09-26) who had just stepped down as chairman of the AAU Physique Committee. The NPC has gone on to become the most successful bodybuilding organization in the U.S., and is the amateur division of the IFBB in the United States. The late 1980s and early 1990s saw the decline of AAU sponsored bodybuilding contests. In 1999, the AAU voted to discontinue its bodybuilding events.(Wikipedia, 2012a)

In the early 2000s, the IFBB was attempting to make bodybuilding an Olympic sport. It obtained full IOC membership in 2000 and was attempting to get approved as a demonstration event at the Olympics which would hopefully lead to it being added as a full contest. This did not happen. Olympic recognition for bodybuilding remains controversial since many argue that bodybuilding is not a sport.(Littman, 2012)

On Labor Day 2006, California governor and seven times Mr. Olympia winner Arnold Schwarzenegger, a Weider protégé, presented him with the Venice Muscle Beach Hall of Fame's Lifetime Achievement award. Schwarzenegger credited Weider with inspiring him to enter bodybuilding and to come to the United States.(Wikipedia, 2012b)

Since the early 1970's bodybuilding had developed the stigma of steroid taking freaks. Due to the growing concerns of the high cost, health consequences and illegal nature of steroids many organizations have formed in response and have deemed themselves "natural" bodybuilding competitions. In addition to the concerns noted, many promoters of bodybuilding have sought to shed the "freakish" reputation that the general public perceives of bodybuilding and have successfully introduced a more mainstream audience to the sport of bodybuilding by including competitors whose physiques appear much more attainable and realistic.(Wikipedia, 2012a)

This book will follow along those lines of developing physiques which appear attainable and realistic. Modern Bodybuilding Techniques are those of a 'natural' bodybuilder and my philosophy and method will give you the reader results of an aesthetically pleasing physique.

Before I go into detail on the techniques of Modern Bodybuilding, we first need to have a brief overview on the workings of the systems of the human body.

The Human Body

An Introduction
The human body can be described as two branches of science. To help you understand your body parts and functions the science explains anatomy and physiology.

Anatomy refers to the study of structure and the relationships among structures. And physiology deals with the functions of the body parts, and how those body parts work.(Gerard Tortora, 1984) Or to put it another way, how we as living organisms perform the various functions of life. Since the two branches cannot be completely separated. Let me go into more detail of how the human body's structures and functions work together.

The human body consists of several levels of structural organization that are associated with one another in several ways. The lowest level or organization, the ***Chemical*** level, includes all chemical substances essential for maintaining life.

The chemicals, in turn, are put together to form the next higher level of organization, which is the ***Cellular*** level. Cells are the basic structural and functional units of an organism.

The next higher level of structural organization is the *Tissue* level. Tissues are made up of groups of similar cells and their intercellular material that perform certain special functions. Cells produce enzymes which are needed to digest proteins. Other examples of tissues in your body are muscle tissue, connective tissue, and nervous tissue.

Different kinds of tissues are joined together to form an even higher level of organization and we call this the *Organ* level. Organs are structures of definite form and function composed of two of more different tissues. Organs can be described as the heart, liver, lings, brain and stomach for example.

At this point I did not want to get too bogged down in the pure science of Anatomy and Physiology as it will fry your brain. But if we take a step back now and focus a bit more on the *Tissue* level I will continue to highlight a few more important things.

Muscle Tissue
Let's start by explaining exactly what muscle is. Muscle is a soft tissue that contains protein filaments which move past each other. This creates a contraction that alters the shape and length of a particular cell. And the function of a muscle is to basically make force and trigger movement. Makes sense right?

Without muscle you wouldn't be able to sit, walk, smile, laugh or even talk!

Muscles help you sit up straight. They are responsible for your movement along with your internal organ movement, like your heart for example! When you eat it's your muscles that are responsible for digesting the food and transforming it into useable energy. So you can see muscle tissue is extremely important for life.

You need healthy muscle tissue to get out of your bed in the morning. To brush your teeth and your hair and to eat your healthy protein and complex carbohydrate balanced breakfast. Which of course you do every morning right?

Now I'm going to get a little more "science-y" on you for a minute because it's important to understand the basics of muscle before we move forward. Your muscles are created specifically from the mesoderm layer of various embryonic germ cells. Muscle tissue is comprised of protein and that is not created or stored long-term by the body. This means that in order to maintain cell structure, grow, build muscle, burn fat, and have energy, you need to eat lean complete protein sources in the proper amount each day. If not, your body will actually revert to breaking down your muscle instead of fat and use it for energy. Definitely not what you want to happen if you are trying to lose weight and build a lean, healthy and sexy body!

The Muscular System
So now we are going to have a look at your muscular system as a whole. Your muscular system is responsible for moving you. And there are approximately 700 labeled muscles attached to your bones; about half of your body weight! Pretty impressive if I do say so myself.

Every one of these muscles is an organ that's made of your skeletal muscle tissue, tendons, blood vessels and various nerves. And did you know that all muscles are not one in the same. There are three main kinds of muscles.

Visceral Muscle

These muscles are located right inside of your intestines, stomach, blood vessels and various other organs. Visceral muscles are the weakest of the bunch and their function is to cause contractions. Just like a woman experiences while giving birth!

Visceral muscles are involuntary because your brain makes sure the contractions take place unbeknown to your conscious awareness. In other words you don't have to think about making your digestive muscles work in order to process your food - good thing!

And I'm sure you've heard of "smooth muscle" being used before. Visceral muscles are commonly called smooth muscle because it looks smooth and uniform if you happen to see it up close. It looks very different in comparison to the other two main types of muscles.

Cardiac Muscle
If you are thinking 'heart' you are bang on here! Cardiac muscles are located only in the heart and their responsibility is to pump oxygenated and nutrient rich blood through your body to all your internal organs and systems. So it makes sense the healthier and stronger you are, the more effectively and efficiently your cardiac muscle will be able to pump.

Lucky for you and me your cardiac muscle can't be controlled by you. It's an involuntary muscle regulated by your unconscious mind. And it's a combination of your hormones and electronic signals from your brain that cause your heart rate to contract at a faster or slower pace. The natural pacemaker of your heart is the catalyst for your other cardiac muscle cells to contract when they are supposed to.

This process is intrinsic and these muscles have both light and dark stripes, otherwise referred to as striated. Do you feel like you're back in biology class yet?

Cardiac muscles are built strong having branched Y and X shaped cells tightly interwoven with unique junctions referred to as intercalated disks. Which are finger-like projections from the nearby cells that bond to make a secure connection between the cells. This helps these cells to stand up to high blood pressure because of the stress of pumping blood through your body. This unit also assists in pushing electrochemical signals swiftly between cells so your heart can beat as one.

Skeletal Muscle
This muscle is the only muscle tissue in your body that is voluntary - meaning you control it consciously. It doesn't matter whether you are running, walking, skipping or dancing. You need your skeletal muscles to do this. If you didn't have them you would just be a puddle of "gunk" on the floor.

Its function is to contract to literally move certain parts of your body closer to the bone in which this muscle is adhered to. In general the majority of your skeletal muscles are hooked up to two bones across a joint. So moving these bones closer together is what this muscle does.

Skeletal muscles are striated just like your cardiac muscle and the fibers are truly strong. And just in case you are wondering why they are called skeletal muscles? It's just because they are always touching your skeleton in at least one spot. Unless maybe you are injured and we don't want to get into that just yet!

Are you still with me? Now we could go on in a lot more detail but I think you've got the gist of things for now. If there's anything else that I need to address to help you understand Anatomy and Physiology I will do so when we run into it.

Let us move on to the next piece of the puzzle, which is the DACT Method and basically the crux of this book. Essentially, the DACT Method is the Decision, Action, Commitment and Today methodology or philosophy of how I pilot my life and hopefully how you adopt this philosophy as well.

Let me expand on this philosophy in a bit more detail below.

The DACT Method

Make a Decision
The first thing you have to do if you want to make a change in your body is to make a decision. You have to decide that you want to take up weight training. You've also got to determine what sort of weight training you'd like to do and to what level you want to get into it. Do you want to make it a career or do you just want to learn how to power lift and go from there?

This means the type of training you are going to do needs to be considered when you are creating your routine or plan of action. In this book we are looking at a muscle building routine that is hypertrophic and looking for maximum muscle gain. This means we will follow a routine setting us up for success with a lean and fabulously muscular body when all is said and done!

Take Action

So after you've decided you are going to build nice big muscles you are going to need to figure out how you're going to get to the finish line. You are going to have to determine what steps you're going take to make it happen. Does this all make sense to you?

Perhaps you're a couch potato and are going to have to first convince yourself to get your lazy butt off the couch, put away the Twinkies and get to the gym for some cardio and weight lifting exercises. You are in charge of you and if YOU don't commit to actually taking action then you aren't going to get results. You can't set yourself up for success if you don't REALLY want it and instead will be blowing a whole lot of hot air, just spinning your wheels.

It's going to take hard work and commitment to get a beautifully sculpted muscular body. If you are willing to accept this and take Action to get it done, then you are one step closer to being jaw dropping "eye-candy!"

Commitment

I hate to burst your bubble, but fabulously ripped bodies don't just happen! People aren't born with it, nor is it easy! If you are drooling over the cute hunk, with a hard packed six pack, drool away. You can bet your ass he works hard to keep it with extremely healthy eating and a training regimen that just might make you cry. It may "appear" easy to do but I'm here to tell you it's not.

If you want that rock hard "eye-candy" body, then you are going to have to Commit to it. You are going to have to take excuses out of your repertoire and commit to training hard and eating right to make it happen. And don't forget that it takes time to make this sort of thing happen. My magic wand has been in the repair shop for quite some time so you are going to have to go about getting into fabulous shape the hard way. And this starts with committing to the pressure of change!

You will need to open your mind to a lifestyle change. Not just for a few weeks but you need to make it manageable and reasonable to maintain for the rest of your life! If you are going to do it, you might as well do it right. Make your positive life habits stick so that you don't have to keep going back through the process. Because each time you try the quick fix here you make it harder for your mind and body to come together. Harder to support any sort of positive lifestyle change that will give you the body you want and all the good that comes with it. Am I making sense here?

Do it Today
This essentially means stop procrastinating! Aren't you tired of waiting for the "perfect" day to get started losing fat and building lean and sexy muscle? Well I am. And this is my book, so you need to get started right now – Do-it-Today!

So today you are going to hit the gym and start training, ditch fast food, make healthy food choices and stop it with your nightly pig-out sessions when you're bored!

You either do it or you don't. But one thing to keep in mind here is not to get too rigid and set in your ways. If you only see black and white you are setting yourself up to fail. You're human right? Good! Whew! So expect you may take a step back here and there. So what! Recognize it - forget about it - and move forward full steam ahead! You will see quickly these minor bleeps in the road really don't affect the big picture so don't use them as an excuse to fail.

DACT is simply another word for SUCCESS. We just haven't got it in the dictionary yet!

Now what I want you to do is this. Firstly, go and grab a piece of A4 blank paper and a permanent marker. Next, write on that piece of paper the following: 'DACT' in the biggest letters that will fit on that piece of paper. Then I want you to stick/place that piece of paper in the most prominent position in your house. Maybe on the fridge, or the wall above the TV or above your bed?

The reason that I want you to do this is because we are going to build a Mantra! A Mantra simply means a sacred utterance, a syllable, word, or group of words believed by some to have psychological and spiritual power.

I want you to look at this piece of paper with the word 'DACT' on it several times a day, and when you see this word, it is the trigger for you to take 'ACTION' and do it 'TODAY'.

Time for you to get to it don't you think? DACT?!

Now that you have the DACT Mantra embedded into you psyche, I am going to teach you the Modern Bodybuilding Techniques that will make you successful in achieving that sculpted body you desire.

Modern Bodybuilding Techniques

How to Exercise
Let's begin by talking about what the definition of exercise is exactly. Exercise is any sort of activity that requires your physical effort, often executed or carried out for a specific purpose, to keep or improve your health and overall fitness capacity. Seems pretty straight forward don't you think?

And the first thing you are going to do to exercise is to get your lazy butt up off the couch and get to release those endorphins of yours! Ok - now what? Well depending your physical health, age and ability, you will exercise different than another person might.

Whether you are going to exercise by walking, riding your bike, gardening, doing some lawn bowling, joining a gym or just running up and down the stairs in your house, here are a few keys to remember.

* Start Slow - It really doesn't matter if you were "Mr. Athlete" twenty years ago or not. If you haven't been off the couch in a few years you are going to need to ease yourself into exercising just to be safe.

* Check In With Your Doctor - It's always important to check with your doctor before you take action on any exercise routine you've decided upon. Better safe than sorry!

* Do It Regularly - Exercising is like a masterpiece in progress. It takes time to get used to and perfect. It will take time for your head and physical body to connect and work as one.

* Practice - Practice makes perfect and you need to stick with exercising if it's going to benefit your overall health. It really doesn't do you very much good to start biking - overdo it and quit a few days later. Or to try moving your body with an aerobics class for a few sessions and then quit. Exercise is only beneficial if you stick with it!

* Diversity - If you are using exercise to help build lean muscle and lose weight, improve energy stores, and deter

free radicals from taking over and to put a permanent smile upon your face: Change it up! Diversity is the key to continuous progress mentally and physically with exercise. It keeps you from getting bored and makes sure different muscles are always being used and this keeps both your mind and body guessing. Burning more calories and moving you closer faster to you weight-loss goals.

So if you have been rowing half the summer for your exercise it's time for you to switch things up to keep seeing results. How about testing out a boot camp class or what about getting a personal trainer to set you up on an intense and challenging program?

How to Work Out
Now that you know the keys behind how to exercise it's time for you to take Action! You need to first commit to exercising and decide how you are going to work-out. Nobody can make you do this. Not your doctor, friends, family or partner. YOU have to decide that you are going to make exercise a routine part of your everyday because that's exactly what your body wants and deserves.

Let's rewind time a few hundred years. Back in the olden day's people didn't need to worry about exercising because they HAD to do it to survive. They didn't have cell phones to ring the nearest pizza delivery outlet whenever they were hungry. They didn't even have fridges to keep milk cold and cheese fresh. They didn't have grocery stores and fast-food joints on every block making food a focus instead of a necessity for survival.

If these people wanted to eat they have to grab their spear or bow and arrow, horse if they were lucky, and head out for a few days or weeks to track down some food. If they happened to find a caribou or buffalo they could outsmart.

Then they were on cloud nine because they knew they could feed their family or tribe for at least a week or so!

So after they physically hunted and killed the caribou they had to drag it two miles back to camp. Then they had to go gather the firewood they would need to cook it. And at some point they would have to also find the natural supplies they would use to make their bowls and eating utensils. By the time they cooked the food and were finished eating, wasting nothing, they had to head back out again for another kill if they wanted to stay strong and survive!

Boy do we have it easy. Point is all this physical DAILY energy is what your body is created to do. And our modern day lazy society has short-circuited our brains and put everything else before the intrinsic and basic needs of your body. Now we have to make a point of exercising an hour each day if we want to keep our health and extend our time here on earth. Does that make sense? We have to think about how we are going to work-out, whereas way back they didn't have to. Workout or die right?

Same sort of thing right now although not as quick usually!

When you are working out you have a focus. You aren't just "moving" around here and there. You are setting a plan in place to reach a goal. So if you are planning to drop twenty pounds to get that nice flat belly or firm round but, you are going to need to set up a workout plan that will set you up for success. One that will help propel you to your goal.

Let's start with the most effective workout and that involves interval training. Building lean muscle and utilizing cardiovascular activity to burn fat faster. And by alternating levels of low intensity with levels of higher exertion you are going to maximize results and minimize time. Does that make sense?

If you are going to train you might as well do it right - right?

You want to make your training effective and efficient. That said here are a few pointers to help you work-out harder, faster and longer.

Fact: When working out at one point or another your mind will drift. Yes, you have the energy to keep going but the receptors in your brain referred to as interleukin-6 interfere. What happens is you actually feel pain before your tank is empty. And what your brain is doing is trying to protect you from injuring yourself and telling your body it's quittin' time! So your psychosomatic is forcing you to stop, not your actual physical ability. Ultimately this stops you from working out longer and getting faster results!

Why You Stop?

Well when your body is running low on glycogen, which is your main muscle fuel source your body will slow down. Fat is also a fuel source but your body neglects to tell you this when your muscles are aching.

Here is where you need to put your mind to work and imagine yourself continuing. If you're running imagine a huge magnet in front of you pulling your forward. It really does work! Or of course you could picture a hot muscle rippling guy or sexy lingerie clad girl just out of reach in front of you and watch your pace pick up instantaneously!

Why You Can't Bench Press Any More?

Here is where you need to set yourself up for success and be specific about it. If you set a casual goal of 6 - 12 reps you aren't likely to hit it. But if you set your goal for three sets of 8 reps you WILL succeed! It's mind over matter folks. Focus on your technique as you're using over 30 muscles for your bench presses and when your muscles tire it's your form that tends to go out the window first. Improper form is dangerous and ineffective!

What Should You Do When You Can't Lift Anymore?

First make sure you have a spotter. Then you should lift more! Dig deep and pull off a few more. Even if they are just half reps, that's more than you did last time. Meaning you're making progress and implementing some forced muscle building that will get you bigger and stronger faster - believe it!

Why Are You Slowing Up On The Cardio?

Well because you're running out of steam my friend!

So How Do You Speed Up?

Well you need to stop and do another cardio activity. Change your focus and implement some interval training. This will give your body the chance to engage different muscles and recharge you just enough to give you the energy you need to keep on trekking." I think I can - I think I can - I think I can." Remember that smart little train? Act like a train and just do it!

If you've been biking and just can't do it anymore then get off and go into a light jog for two minutes. Pick up the pace to a sprint for a minute and then drop to the floor for ten pushups. Immediately after, squeeze off twenty crunches and ten "burpees". Take a ten second breather and then repeat the process. The idea is to keep your mind and body guessing with intense and effective interval training to finish off your training session in style and strong!

I think you get the idea here. You need to make the most of your workout sessions and always push yourself for a little more. Keep things diverse and effective and never let your mind tell you there's nothing left. Dig deep because you know and I know you can always do one or two more!

Where to Train
Well most bodybuilders use a gym facility for their training that's equipped with plenty of free weights, weight machines and cardiovascular equipment. Now you can pull a "Rocky" and look to find a farm and do a little innovative work there but that one is a little bit tougher to implement!

Most places have a wide arrange of gyms from which to choose so what you'll likely want to do is find the one that suits you best. A few factors to consider are:

- Hours of operation
- Size of the facility
- Equipment
- Cost
- Instructors
- Location
- Atmosphere

You don't want to join a gym that is only open from 7-5 if that's your work day! Good thing most gyms have long hours and some are even 24 hours which is even better, especially if you work shift. This just means you can get into a routine that works for you and this means you are more likely to stick with it. Did you know that if you do something for at least 8 weeks you can consider it a habit?

And only you know you. So it's important the gym you choose is large enough for you. If you aren't good with enclosed spaces and a gym always seems to be crowded and small, you are better to look elsewhere. Don't give yourself a reason not to come right off the bat!

Of course the gym you choose needs to have adequate equipment. And the majority of gyms more than accommodate here. So you want to make sure there are plenty of free weights and weight machines because that's going to be where a lot of your focus is.

And if you're on a budget you are going to have to make sure the gym you choose is affordable for you. Don't go for a high end gym if you can't afford it. That just doesn't make sense. Find one that you can comfortably pay for so that financial constraints don't cause interference with your goals.

Most bodybuilders have a coach at one point or another so before you sign on the dotted line you are going to need to meet with a few of them and see if you connect. There is no use joining a gym if you aren't comfortable with the staff. That's just a means to an end. If you are going to be successful in you quest to build a spectacularly sculpted body you need to be certain you've got support in place that works for YOU!

And you'd be surprised how many people don't take into consideration where this facility is located before committing. If you work long days and decide on a gym that's out of your way, a good half hour from your house, you're looking for trouble. Ask yourself if you are really going to trek out of your way to go? This just doesn't make sense, especially if there is another closer to your home. Depending on when you are planning to hit the gym, you want one close to your house or work. The one that makes it most convenient to get too even when you don't want to go.

If you actually have to drive right by it on the way home even better! Makes it a little tougher for you to not bother when it's right in your face. This is especially important if you're pressed for time. I'm pretty sure you get the gist of what I'm squabbling about here!

Another factor to consider is the overall atmosphere. If you walk into the facility and feel like you are way out of place or just get a bad vibe, you can do a few things.

* Relax and give yourself a chance to blend in. Many people take time to get comfortable in their surroundings and you need to be aware of this. And chances are pretty good you might also just be looking for any old excuse not to get started. Could this be true?

If so give yourself a smack on the butt and get good with the facility!

* Try another. If there are just too many little things that bother you and you know you won't be able to ever get comfortable then you're going to have to find another place to train. And if this is the only place around then you are going to have to decide how badly you want to get lean and sexy. If you REALLY want it then nothing should stand in your way - think "Rocky!"

So when you've taken the time to do a little investigative research here hopefully you've come to a decision. Because if you don't have a great place to train, you are selling yourself short here. Set yourself up for success and that's exactly what you'll achieve!

When to Train
This may seem like a no-brainer but looks can be deceiving. A few factors you need to look at here are when you are truly at your best during the day both physically and mentally. You need to look at your own circadian rhythm here.

Are you a morning person or a night owl?

I'll call you a "Lark" if you are one of those annoyingly happy people the moment your eyes open from a deep winter's sleep. Your natural sleep cycle and body rhythm dictates this just may be the best time for you to take advantage of your muscle building ability. After you've had a nice healthy breakfast of course, because running your tank on empty, especially when you are training hard is a seriously stupid move!

Now if you're an "Owl" and seem to come alive when the sun goes, you might do well making sure your training sessions are later in the day or at night. Of course this has to work with your work schedule too.

Suffice to say, the majority of the population falls somewhere in between the two. Which means you can pretty much workout any time of the day you choose and be effective. You know you here my friend so all you need to figure out is what works best for you!

And just for fun here are a few factors that support different times in training throughout the day.

First Thing in the Morning
- This is when testosterone is running high
- Now is when you are cognitively sharp and your memory is working best

Early Afternoon
- This is when your endorphins mask pain the best
- Your adrenaline and energy are usually rising as the afternoon progresses

Evening
- Here is when your agility and temperature peak
- You are mentally strong, physically strong and your lungs are at their best

Late Evening
- Here is where your melatonin or sleep drug start to increase in production
- Your bodily processes are getting ready to shut down for the night

Bottom line is there are always exceptions to the rules. You need to look at your daily schedule and when you feel most energetic. This is likely the best time for you to hit the gym and get pumping!

What to Wear
NO SHIRT, NO SHOES, NO SERVICE!

For some the smaller the better! What I'm going to tell you is you need to be comfortable and make sure you don't make others uncomfortable. Remember everyone is there training hard and trying to stay focused on what they are doing - not you!

For most weight lifters this is the gear they need.

- Shorts
- T-shirt
- Good Shoes

Again the idea is to get comfortable so you can stop concentrating on what you're wearing and get focused on lifting weights! Most guys go for the shorts and t-shirt thing. Some do muscle shirts, others really tight t-shirts and some wear just a plain old ratty shirt. It really doesn't matter so long as most of your chest is covered.

You're not here to show off or hide for that matter. You are at the gym to train and better your body - period!

Now I would like to talk a little about weight belts if I may. Many weight lifters DO NOT use a weight belt because this does give you a false sense of security and often allows your technique to be less than perfect.

You will not injure yourself if you aren't lifting too heavy and if you are using proper technique. A weight belt really doesn't help unless maybe you've already suffered from a back injury. Be very careful here because many lifters assume that just because they are sporting one of those big-ass weight belts that they are "safe" from injury.

This couldn't be further from the truth. And one thing you don't want to fool around with is a back injury because of using a weight belt! Are you following?

When you advance from a virgin weight lifter to the serious stuff, you may feel you need a big "honkin" belt. Just be sure you are using one for the "right" reasons. Not just announcing to the world you are pumping iron. And don't pretend you don't know what I'm talking about.

Bottom line is you need to be comfortable. And of course you don't want to look like a knob or not have the proper attire. Oh and I better scoot back to the shoe thing for a minute. I can't stress how important it is to have quality shoes to exercise in. Doesn't matter if you are burning it up on the cardio machines, or grunting it out with some forced reps.

GOOD SHOES ARE A MUST!

Make sure they fit property for your foot. And if you've got ginormous feet - lucky you! - A trip to a custom design expert may be a smart move. Treat your feet with kindness so they will last you a lifetime. Cuz you're screwed if you wear them out early!

Exercise Form
You might as well hang your shoes up and not even bother if you aren't willing to make CERTAIN your form is correct in any and all weight lifting you do. Is that clear enough for you!

Think of it like springboard diving in the Olympics. Who wins? The athlete with the BEST form. If they don't have very good form they will fail in their Olympic dreams and they might embarrass themselves with a big fat belly-flop during the competition.

In race car driving the stakes are a little higher. If you lose focus and waver off your technically accurate race you might very well get carted off the track in a body bag! No joke!

Well the same principle applies to exercise from although maybe not so severely. If you want results you're going to have to practice elite form. This doesn't mean PERFECT but it does mean good. And you should always be working on your technique and form because the more precision you have here the better off you will be.

Your body will get hunky faster and you aren't going to create or awaken any aches and pains that just might spoil your parade. I can't count all the times I've watched some young "hunk-wanta-be" lifting too much weight and using improper form. First of all, they are probably wreaking their back, and secondly, they aren't going to get results for their efforts. It's just not going to happen!

Here are a few factors to consider and pay attention to when lifting weights or even stepping on the stepper to get your heart pitter pattering.

Technical Form
I don't care who you are or what level you are training at. You MUST have great technical and precise form when exercising. This means you need to work on keeping your head up and eyes forward when executing squats. You need to make sure you aren't hunched over when climbing away on the stair master. When you are lunging make sure your back is straight and that your shoulders are square, that you are focusing on your breathing and not rushing.

I could go on forever and a day here. But don't worry, I won't. You just need to take the time to consciously remind yourself of everything you should be paying attention for every single rep of every single exercise you do.

When you are tired and near the end of your sets this is going to take even more concentration to execute. Practice might not make perfect but you can get pretty dam close!

And as always it's best to work with a professional initially to make sure you are on track with your technical. Even if you are, it doesn't hurt to check in with one from time to time. This is only going to tweak what you already know. Sounds great to me, how about you?

Boundaries
Everybody has limitations and it's important to recognize them. There is no use crying over the fact that you can't execute a technically correct squat because you have issues with your knees. Maybe you have a boundary because of your knee troubles and have to do half squats instead.

ACCEPT THIS AND MOVE FORWARD!

Work on perfecting your technique with your half squats and quit your crying. Focus on what you can do not what you can't. Acknowledge your boundaries and don't push them. If you ignore them or try anyway, you are going to end up hurting yourself. And if you end up side-lined because of stupidity you are guaranteed not to progress. Make sense to you?

Weight Limitations
It's important that you understand the necessity of starting off slow with the weight lifting and progressing forward as your body and mind allow. Don't be one of those "Dorko's" - that struts into the gym to try and impress the lady's lifting double the weight he should. UGH! I can guarantee you his form sucks and that means he is only hurting his body, rather than building the beautiful sexy rock hard muscles he wants!

Lifting too much weight is probably the number one cause of injury in the gym. And what people don't seem to understand is that when you injure yourself it's VERY hard to ever get your body back to where it was. Injuries don't ever really go away. Sure you'll usually heal in time, but really what happens is your injuries just go to sleep for a while.

Trust me. When you're older they will wake up and make it that much harder to lift the weights you want and stick with it. Do you see where I'm coming from?

Be safe and start WAY light. Make sure you have the right form and practice it so much that it becomes habit. This way when you are challenging yourself with the weight you won't have to literally "think" about technique so much. Yes, you will always have to be aware but the more you learn to become habit the better.

Body Health
Your overall body health also needs to be taken into consideration when you are figuring out your technique. This means if you are a bag of damaged goods. Meaning you have all sorts of injuries to deal with both past and present. Then you need to be extra careful that you are using a technique that accommodates YOUR body condition. An expert will definitely be able to help you here. So maybe you don't have full mobility in your right arm. So modifications in your technical execute may have to be put in place when you are doing biceps curls.

A qualified trainer will be able to help you personalize your technique if that's what your body needs.

And when it comes to the cardio exercise, take note. If you've got bad hips, it doesn't matter how good your technique is when running. Running is NOT an exercise you should be doing. Accept your limitations and maybe opt to work on your technical accuracy in biking or swimming. Work on the muscles that aren't going to hinder you physically. Less stress may be necessary in certain areas and an expert training will be able to tell you exactly what you can and can't do with reference to your current body health.

I hope you're listening here because you want to get your body smoking hot right? Not end up restricting your mobility further. Use your head - your big head here!

Proper form needs to be front and center when you're stretching, weight training, walking/running or doing yoga.

You are looking for progress and proper technique is necessary for progress. Your other option is injury. Even when you are stretching you need to be certain you aren't overextending or rushing through them. This means that you need to take your time to stretch correctly and ensure you are paying attention to your form on each and every stretch. This will warm your muscles up properly and ensure you don't strain your muscles and that you get the results you want.

Ready, set, go!

Training Tempo
This is something that is often ignored when it comes to training. Many weight lifters are more worried about how much they are lifting instead of 'how' they are lifting and at what tempo.

If bigger and better is your goal you need to focus on the tempo!

I'm sure you've seen it when people whip through their routine paying ZERO attention to tempo. That's all fine and dandy but I can tell you they aren't maximizing their muscle building. If fact the opposite is true.

By slowing down the tempo and paying attention to your form, you won't lift as much weight as you do when using momentum.

BUT

You will hit your goals faster! So set your ego aside and slow the pace for the sake of progress.

Training Tempo 101

We'll start with the basics my friend. So please excuse me here if you're a veteran in this weight lifting stuff!

One thing for certain is you NEVER want to weight train at a tempo that doesn't allow for you to lift your weights in a controlled and smooth motion. This means NO SWINGING and NO JERKY MOVEMENTS!

Slow and steady wins the race my friends and if anyone tells you otherwise they don't know what the hell they are talking about!

If you want to be successful with your modern bodybuilding you need to use smooth and controlled motion - PERIOD!

If you are lifting too fast your momentum will take over and this means your muscles aren't working optimally. And more importantly, fast lifting will lead to jerky motions and this will ultimately lead to injury. Sometimes seriously enough delay your progress considerably. And you don't want that right?

Most people refer to tempo as counts. You extend to the count of five and contract to the count of five. Slow and controlled, feeling your muscles, focusing on them while you are lifting.

So let's look at an example here. If you are using 5/0/3 on your squat, it means you will lower to the count of five. No pausing at the bottom, and extend yourself back up in a controlled motion to the count of three. Are you following?

This tempo business also gives you something to focus on, which makes you able to pay more attention to your form and not the clock. Rushing WILL NOT do your body any good whatsoever. And if you are in the habit of zipping through your routine, SHAME ON YOU! Work with a trainer to help them help you break this unproductive habit, so you can get the results you want quickly!

If you are looking to build muscle, a general range of tempo is as follows:
- 2-5 Count on the Eccentric or Negative (lowering/contracting)
- 0-1 Count on the Bottom
- 1-3 Count on the Concentric or Positive (raising/extending)

What's also critical is switching it up regularly. If your body memorizes your tempo, it will start to get lazy. This means your results will plateau. By changing your tempo you will keep your body and mind thinking and this is exactly what you need to do to maximize your results!

Also, by pausing at the bottom of an exercise, you're removing all momentum and this really challenges your muscles in the concentric or upward motion. Normally you don't pause at the top of an exercise unless you are doing specialty breathing sets for training.

Have you ever heard of QUICK LIFTING? It's often done specifically for strength training competitions or when athletes are being tested and evaluated. This is NOT an effective route for building your body big and strong with muscle. This type of lifting occurs when individuals go for the highest number of repetitions without worrying about form or technique.

In other words it's simply a measure for neural ability and endurance of your muscles. It's useless for pointing your body in the direction of muscle building. Unfortunately this kind of training often results in avoidable injury.

If you want to up your tempo the odd time for variety, you'll do well with using the count 1/0/1. This is extremely different than the counts our body is used to, and it will help to maximize your workouts by making your muscles think.

RED ALERT! Keep in mind you never want to lift so fast that you are out of control. This just means you are an accident waiting to happen.

Breathing Tempo

In basic, you should inhale during your eccentric portion of your exercise and exhale while hitting the concentric part. So with a squat you would be inhaling while lowering yourself and exhaling while rising up.

To keep it simple, you take a deep breath in just prior to lift off and continue on from there. One FULL breath with each rep.

Yes, you were born breathing - hopefully anyway! But when training, this will take some time to get used to. You will have to concentrate on your breathing technique for the first while. One thing for certain is you don't want to develop crappy breathing habits. Things like holding your breath are a definite no-no. Not unless you want to go to "PassOutVille!"

Holding your breath will increase your blood pressure and stress out your internal ticker. And there are weight trainers that believe they get a little extra push doing this.

Don't! It's dumb and will wear your out faster. Your mind and muscles need oxygen to perform. Never forget it!

Now there is one exception to this rule and that comes with Static Contraction Weight Training Methods and Slow Lifting. But only with experts that know exactly what they're doing. The 30 seconds of holding your breath can be too long to sustain you in a stressful situation. Please take note that steady and controlled breathing take the gold medal here.

Bottom line is, work on breathing properly so you aren't going to steal energy from your muscles and hinder your performance.

Rest Intervals - Critical

When you are looking to pump iron to build your sexy muscles strong, normally resting 2-3 minutes between sets is just about perfect.

What does the rest do?

Well it gives your muscles the ability to recover and get fully energized for the next pounding. Makes sense the more they're recovered, the more weight they will be eager to handle.

So what is circuit training? It's not effective for building muscle. Essentially the goal here is to scoot from exercise to exercise. Making this an anaerobic and aerobic training session. Great for getting you into shape but not so great for building your body muscle strong!

Of course varying your time between sets is beneficial with maximizing your muscle building sessions. And yes, you will be making the right move if you shock your system from time to time. Try minimizing your rest time between sets. Throw the unexpected at your body from time to time and you will be rewarded!

Use it or lose it my friends!

It's also important to note that compound exercises will take longer to recover from than simple isolated ones. Although it's important to keep your rest periods the same for rhythmic purposes.

So what should you do during your rest periods? Call your mom, text your girlfriend or grab a sandwich! KIDDING! It's important you stay focused on your exercise routine from start to finish. So why not get your mind actually visualizing your next weight lifting move while stretching lightly between sets?

The last thing you want to do is start thinking about groceries, work problems or the last fight you had with your partner. Just don't let your head go there!

Use a Timer

Don't trust your head to measure time accurately. There's a HUGE difference between my "steamboats" and yours. Use a clock or stopwatch to make certain you stay on schedule. Your mind is incredibly sneaky and powerful, and it will trick you if you let it!

Changing it Up

Routine and the same tempo are nice. We are creatures of habit and naturally find comfort in routine. But what you are doing in the gym is trying to get your muscles and body to react. And by doing the same thing over and over again you just aren't going to react.

If you know that an annoying co-worker is going to ask you out every Friday night, eventually you just aren't even going to react when he asks you. Well the same thing applies with weight training. If you don't change your routine and tempo, your body will memorize your routine and exert only the exact amount of energy required. It will get lazy, and lazy doesn't get you maximum results.

To get results you need to get your psychosomatic working. You need to keep your body and mind thinking always. Minor changes yield maximum results.

Each of these factors is necessary in maximizing your results. Just remember, tempo plays a huge role in your muscle building success!

Starting Weights
Building muscle by lifting weights is fantastic for burning fat, getting "Hulkster" strong and keeping your bones

strong at any age. Whatever your reasoning, weight lifting is a fantastic move!

LEAVE YOUR EGO AT THE DOOR!

Consider this point one. If your ego gets in the way here you will end up embarrassed at some point for getting stuck with the freakin barbell on your neck! Or you are going to seriously get knocked down a few notches by getting injured.

None of which are worth it. And what should really piss you off if is they're both totally avoidable!

Be smart and be safe, and you'll be good to go.

Alright, here are a few more pointers to get you started.

Ask and you shall receive!

Make sure you know how to use the machines BEFORE you start. So ask QUALIFIED people how to use each machine. Most are happy to help, because form is incredibly important here. Most good gyms offer a few free training sessions to get you set up on a program. Something to consider when you are choosing your training facility.

And if you need to hire a trainer to learn the basics - DO IT! It is imperative that you know what you're doing before you start training.

Your muscles build strong when you're resting, not training.

Maybe this is a shocker for you and maybe not. Either way it's a cold hard fact. It's so crucial to rest your separate muscle groups after training them hard. What happens is your muscles rebuild depending on how hard your work them. When you are training your muscles you essentially are damaging them, so your body will repair them stronger than before. This means bigger and better, and that's all good for you.

So it makes sense to alternate muscle groups. And it's logical to ensure you've got a few days each week for full rest. This will maximize your performance and results.

Fueling your body right.

Your body needs adequate vitamins and minerals on a regular basis if you expect it to build beautiful strong muscles. You need to get plenty of protein, carbs and good fat to build your body strong. Supplementation is also a wise move when you getting serious about weight training.

In fact, if you don't give your body enough protein on a regular basis it will actually start using the muscle you already have for energy. The problem is that your body can't make protein and it doesn't store it. AND it needs protein to build muscle. So if you aren't giving your body complete protein sources before and after muscle training you are going to be up "Crap Creek without a paddle!"

And a complete protein is found mainly in lean meat options. With the only non-meat complete protein being quinoa. Most plant protein sources are incomplete and need to be in combination with one another to be complete. Of course different bodies absorb different combinations better, so other protein sources are a gamble at best.

Fueling your mind and body right is essential for building your body strong and muscular. It will be important for you to get your carbs and protein, especially before and after your training. A small snack works great to keep your energy levels up for the challenge. And of course you can restore your energy stores after your workout too.

Slow out of the starting gates.

Sure you are likely eager to get your body ripped. But honestly folks, slow and steady wins the race. It's wise to start off with light weights until you get used to the muscles you are using. Don't challenge your muscles right off the bat. You want to feel the burn in each muscle group, so that you know exactly what you're doing when you hit the heavier weights. This isn't going to happen by waving your magic wand. You're going to have to work at it and stop yourself and make the adjustments necessary to learn how to make your muscles work.

Patience pays off!

Progressive Advancement

Successful weight training means constantly improving. Pushing yourself after every exercise to do more. This doesn't necessarily mean lifting more but it does mean doing more. Maybe you are going to add one more rep on your bench press or put another pound or two on your weighted lunges.

If you keep doing the same weight, at the same tempo, with the same number of reps EVERY week, YOU ARE NOT PROGRESSING. This means you are not building your muscles big and strong.

ALWAYS challenge yourself to do a touch more at every single workout. This is going to push your mind and body, and you are going to get ripped results. Sound good to you?

Try Full Body Three Times a Week

Part of starting slow with your weight training is for the process of learning. So it makes sense that you train your FULL body three times a week to start. Rather than splitting it up into specific muscle groups just yet. So start off with light weights doing legs, chest, back, arms, abs etc. every workout.

This gives you a chance to get your body accustom to training and recognizing how each muscle works.

Accountability

Many people have a tough time getting their butt out of bed for a hard workout unless they have someone to answer to. It doesn't matter if it's a workout partner, a trainer or a friend. It just seems to be human nature to be okay with letting ourselves down. But it's a different story when you've got someone to face if you decide to get lazy and hit the snooze button instead of pumping iron. I think you know what I'm talking about.

You know you, and you need to ensure the measures are in place to make your muscle building program succeed. Just do it!

How Many Reps
Okay before we get to this you need to understand what REPs and SETs mean. A rep or repetition is a complete motion of an exercise. And simply put a set is a group of consecutive repetitions.

So if you did three sets of eight reps for your squats. It means you did eight consecutive squats, three times.

And the number of reps you do depends on the experience level you're at and your goals. If you are looking to build big muscle, then you're going to want to do fewer reps with heavier weights. This forces your muscles to maximize energy output fast and exhaust themselves fast.

If on the other hand you are looking to tone your body sleek. You'll want to do lots of reps with lighter weights. So maybe 12 - 15 reps of 3 sets. If you use weights that are ultra-light you won't gain any strength because your muscles aren't stressed enough to get strong.

IMPORTANT NOTE: When you are lifting weights to build muscle strength you should be struggling to lift the last two or three reps of each set. And of course you should be able to pound off fewer reps with each set if you are really pounding away. This means you are forcing your muscles to perform when your body is telling you to stop. Mind over matter. You'll understand this after a few months of weight training.

Many successful weight lifters will alternate heavy and lighter days just to keep the muscles guessing. This will help you build strength and improve your endurance some.

In general you'll use heavier weights to for your larger muscles; back, chest and thighs. And of course lighter weights for your shoulders, abs and arms. Experiment and find the weights that suit you best. Also fool around with your reps until you find the number that clicks.

It's also very important to write down what amount of weight you are using for specific exercises and how many reps and sets you are pumping off. This way you aren't left guessing if you're progressing forward or not. You will have it in black and white.

Now when it comes to the number of sets that are most effective, you are going to hit a brick wall. There are conflicting bouts of information here. Some experts argue that one heavy set does just as much muscle building as three. Particularly for the first few months of training.

If you are just starting, one set is fine and just make sure you're feeling it on the last two or three reps. If you've been doing 8 reps for a few sessions and find that you aren't being challenged anymore then you need to increase your weight. This will make it challenging and progressive. It means you are getting strong muscles and are well on your way to reaching your goals.

Now if you are really lifting heavy you should have a spotter so that you can push past and through your limitations. In other words you'll go until your muscle literally fails on you. Something you need to gets lots of experience first before it becomes part of your training session.

Just think of it as something to look forward to!

After 2-4 weeks a beginner will generally start to slowly increase their weights. Listen to your body but always look to challenge yourself. If you're serious about building muscle you'll progress fairly quickly.

Breaking Your Muscles In

It's just like breaking in a new baseball glove or braking in your new leather shoes. If you dive right in full force you will pay for it. Same thing goes with your muscles. Slow and steady wins the race and taking the time to break your muscles in is what smart people do. And you are a smart cookie right?

A few factors to consider are:
- Eating Right
- Stretching
- Light Weights First
- Tender Loving Care
- Listen To Your Body

Eating Right

Your body and mind are interconnected and you need to fuel your body "right" if you are going to build your body right. Start by eating a good breakfast and eat regular mini-meals throughout the day to keep your energy stores up and blood sugar level.

Like it or not your internal health is going to dictate how efficiently your body is going to build muscle. EAT right and you will do well!

Stretching

Stretching is critical in any exercise routine. And when you're trying to break your muscles in the more you can improve your mobility and flexibility the better. Stretching your muscles before, during and after your training sessions will help your muscles grow. By expanding the surface area of your muscles you are increases that size they can be. Stretching will also help ensure more essential vitamins, minerals and oxygenated blood gets to your muscles and this means you can perform longer and with a higher intensity than you would otherwise.

It also lowers the chances of injuring yourself tremendously. And if you're injured it's pretty tough to build your muscles strong.

Light Weights First

Easy out of the starting gate okay? By starting with light weights you will be able to teach your muscles the expectations, you have without paying the painful price that comes with overdoing it.

You don't have to feel so sore after training that you can hardly roll your butt out of bed. It doesn't have to hurt every step you take, and every move that you make. Yes there will be some days when you push yourself past your limitations and your body reminds you of this with some soreness. That's okay.

Just understand you don't have to take the painful route when you start off. Slow and steady wins the race. Your muscles will thank you for it.

Tender Loving Care

Be nice to your body through this transition. Take a bath after a workout or get a massage to help your muscles recover and relax. You need to take the time to teach your muscles what your new expectations are going to be. A little tender loving care definitely doesn't hurt!

Listen To Your Body

Very rarely in life do we listen to our body. Now you've got to start listening. If you overdo it one day with the weights, take it easy the next day. This doesn't mean you get a free class to skip muscle building. But it does mean you have the right to knock it back a few notches for a moment or two.

The more you tune into your body and the needs it makes obvious, the more it's going to trust you and perform.

Each of these factors are going to help your muscles ease nicely into your new muscle building routine, and this means you are going to get sexy buff quicker. Nothing wrong with that!

Progression
In order to make change, as humans we need to be able to measure progress. We need to be able to actually see our success. That our efforts are matching our results. Because if we don't get this reassurance we will allow our self-destructive egos to get in the way and permit the "change" from happening.

I don't want to go all psychology on you but that's the basics of it.

Think about it for a minute. If you are trying to get over your fear of heights you are going to want to see that the little steps you are taking are progressive. Maybe you have been so afraid to face this fear that you haven't even mustered up the courage to go upstairs. An extreme example I know but it will serve to make my point!

So the first day you might gather the courage to step up one step and that may be all you can handle. No matter how small the progress you can "see" that you have progressed.

And the next day you may make it up two more stairs and so on. And it won't be long for you to make it to the very top of the stairs and jump for joy at your successful progress!

YEAH - YOU!

So Progress is critical if you want to have a successful life. If not you would just stay put forever and ever. A factor in progress though is change, and many people fear this. We are naturally creatures of habit and get comfortable and feel safe in our routine. Opposed to change in other words.

Think way, way back to your first day of school. This was a HUGE change for you and it definitely was progress. You may have cried your eyes out the first few days, but eventually you adapted to this change and took a ginormous step forward in your life progressively.

With progress you must open your mind to newness and make adjustments. And it's natural to be freaked out over change. It means you are taking risks, and with risks is the chance of failure. Nobody wants to fail.

Progress is a must in every aspect of life because our world is in constant motion, always changing. Successful progress often happens in small steps. Not rushed or jumped into.

So when it comes to bodybuilding it is important that you progress forward each and every day. Progress needs to happen with regards to:
- Nutrition
- Time Weight Training
- Weight Training Technique
- Weight Training Weight Amounts
- Overall Knowledge about Weight Training

- Attitude and Dedication to Weight Training

If is critical you program yourself to progress in all of the above areas if you are going to succeed in your weight training quest. It's a multi-factorial project that isn't mutually exclusive, but rather collectively exhaustive. You will need to learn to address ALL areas of health and wellness and specifically weight training in order to reach your goals and beyond. In order to progress forward indefinitely and have a beautifully sculpted body of muscle to show for it.

How does that sound to you?

And you can start by writing down your progress. Write down the exercises you are doing and the weight amounts you are using. Also put down the number of sets and reps and what days you are doing this.

Keep a detailed journal of your daily progress because this tool will help to propel you forward ferociously. You will SEE results and want more because your hard efforts are paying off.

Is this making sense?

It's also important to ensure you've got support systems in the loop. If you have a personal trainer great. Maybe you lift with a group or have friends and family that are in your corner cheering you along. Having these external supports are going to ensure your progress is earned and that it sticks, always moving forward.

Mental Factors
Mind over matter my friends!

Whether you are ready to admit it or not the mental factor in weight training is just as important, if not more than the actual physical lifting! If your head isn't in the game your body will not perform. It's as simple as that.

So let's say you're getting frustrated because you've hit a plateau in your weight training. Your efforts are not progressing you forward and you're getting royally ticked off!

Chances are pretty good that your mind is throwing a brick wall in front of you. And when you take control of your thinking and use it positively you will be able to lift more.

If you BELIEVE you can lift it you will. It's your mind that throws a wrench into the equation.

Here are a few strategies to help you get your head on straight and your muscles building beautifully.

When training don't ever think about how heavy the dumbbells are. If you do, your head will signal to your muscles to tell them not to get hurt. Which is what happens when you build muscle through weight lifting. Not a bad thing, but if you don't intercept this message it will interfere with your progress.

Maybe you just want to call it self-sabotage. We always seem to be trying to do it!

Sure there's logic to be had here and you probably do know your limits. But don't bring them into the gym with you. Leave them at the door and focus on doing it. Not the amount of the weights but just doing it.

Maybe you're concerned about injury? Fair enough. But I stand strong in the belief that if you ALWAYS use proper form you will be safe and it doesn't really matter how much you are lifting!

Remember, change is stress to your body and your body really truly hates change. It will do anything, including sabotaging your efforts to keep change from happening.

DAMN YOU BODY!

What you need to do is keep the positive in your mind. When you are executing sets literally TELL your brain how freakin easy this is. Convince yourself it is easy and you will lift more and for longer. And when you hit your failing point your muscles really aren't tired. It's just your nervous system communicating to you to stop because it doesn't want to take ANY chances. It doesn't even want to walk across the street even if you've looked both ways because there is risk. WUSS!

This default mechanism will always be there but you can practice ignoring this and when you do you will strong arm your mind past this pre-set limitation and progress forward happily.

Let me tell you something. You will always have to battle your brain. And when you really can't do any more, all you need to do is 'fake' that you are. Show your brain that you don't have to listen to it and you will get big beautiful sexy muscles faster.

Even if you are just doing a quarter of the fake rep, your brain sees that as you doing it. You are defying it and forcing it to up your pre-set limitations. Does this make sense?

Raising the bar on which you're going to build and now you can truly believe the sky is the limit. And maybe even a little bit higher than this!

Training Partners
It is really tough for many people to create a program and stick to it. Again it's everything else in life getting in the way, and of course your brain working around the clock trying to inhibit change from happening.

Well by having a training partner you are going to better chances at pushing through this barrier, and building your body big, strong and sexy, sexy, sexy! Not to mention the fact that humans need connective relationships to function normally. Nobody wants to be the odd duck on the pond and nobody wants to be left out. We naturally seek companionship in one form or another. This gives us a better shot in battling change.

Even if you are an individual that seems to like some alone time, the chances are pretty good that you would rather weight train with a partner. Birds of a feather flock together! With a partner you will push yourself further because it's not just your own expectations on the table. And it's a heck of a lot more fun!

One thing that often happens when training on your own is that you will cut corners. But with a partner this just won't happen. You will stay focused and on track, working harder each and every session to reach your goals.

And something that's really important to acknowledge is you should train with someone that is close in goals with you. If you try partnering up with your roommate that is only looking to tone up a little and is pretty lax about his training schedule, this isn't going to help you progress forward. Does this sound familiar?

You will want to train with someone that will challenge you and help you grow in the process. Someone that will drive you right past your limitations, inspiring you to want more.

Here are a few qualities you will want to have in a training partner.

ON TIME

Having a training partner that doesn't make excuses is key. They should ALWAYS be there on time. Never missing a workout unless they are sick or a REAL emergency comes up. Excuses are easy, and they are often the kill shot for weight training.

QUALIFIED TO SPOT

If is critical that your training partner knows how to spot you correctly. Having a good spotter will help you to push past your limitations. A peace of mind, and the ability to know that you have someone to watch your back when you go a little too far.

If your spotter is busy with his cell phone or ogling the chicks in the gym while you're pumping iron, you need to toss them out to the curb with the trash!

DISCIPLINE

Trust me on this one. You want a partner that will stick to the plan. Steering off course is just too easy. Make a plan and implement it!

MOTIVATES

An awesome training partner will motivate you to do more. They will push all the right buttons and get you hot and heavy for progress. Your trainer should make you want more all the time. If you've got this then you've just struck gold my friend!

Warm-up and Cool-down
So many people fail when looking to build muscle because they jump right in and don't bother warming up or cooling down. Let me ask you something. Do you warm your car up before you drive it? Do you warm your woman up before you pleasure her? I think you get what I'm saying here.

If you do this you will improve your athletic performance, increase your recovery speed and decrease the risk of ripping a muscle and sidelining yourself.

To start, you need some dynamic stretches with slow and controlled movements through your full range of motions. Stretching isn't a race! It's not something you allot five minutes for and zip right through. Shame on you if you do!

WARM UP POINTERS

- 5-10 minutes of light jogging or other aerobic exercise.
- At least 10 minutes of dynamic stretching - this will reduce muscle stiffness.
- At least 5-10 minutes of getting your head focused on your session and bouncing around a little to accomplish this.

Now you are ready to pump some iron!

ADVANTAGES OF WARMING YOUR MUSCLES AND MIND UP!

- You'll increase the speed of contraction and relaxation of your warmed up muscles
- Deep stretching will reduce muscle stiffness and increase performance
- More oxygen will be available because hemoglobin is responsible for releasing more easily when muscle temperature is higher
- Nerve impulses and muscle metabolism works better at higher temperatures
- Blood flow and circulation will speed up and this means more energy to your muscles for use
- Gets your heart rate up to burn energy and build muscle
- Gets your head focused and ready to train

Now let's move onto the cool down. Which is important because it signals to your tired body that you are done, and it's now time for it to start building muscle!

COOL DOWN POINTERS

- At least 5-10 minutes of jogging/walking - lower body temperate and filter waste from muscles
- At least 5-10 minutes of static stretching

Static Stretches are key to your cool down because they help you muscles chill and relax, realign your muscle fibers and regain their normal motion range. Hold these stretches for at least ten seconds.

BENEFITS OF A PROPER COOL DOWN

- Will help get rid of body waste - inclusive of lactic acid buildup
- Lowers the potential for DOMS (Delayed Onset Muscle Sorenes)
- Decreases the chances of getting dizzy or fainting
- Lowers adrenaline levels
- Brings your heart rate back down to normal

So you can see how critical it is to make certain you establish warm up and cool down habits whenever you train. If you don't you are playing Russian roulette and just might get burned big time!

Stretching
We've touched on this a little above. But expanding here is a good thing. Dynamic Stretching means you are using controlled leg and arm swings that take you gently to the doorstep of your natural limitations of motion. You don't want to do Ballistic Stretching because this means you are pushing a body part past its pre-set limitation.

With dynamic stretching you won't bounce or jerk-off - I mean you won't have any jerky movements! These stretches should be done in sets of 8-15 reps and make sure you stop if you're feeling tired. If your muscles are fatigued they will have less elasticity and this decreases their range of motion altogether.

A FEW EXERCISES:

JOINT ROTATION

Stand with your arms comfortable dangling by your sides, flex, extend and rotate the following joints:

- Wrists and Fingers
- Shoulders and Elbows
- Neck and Trunk
- Hips, Knees and Ankles
- Toes and Feet

NECK

* For flex and extension tuck your chin toward your chest and lilt your chin up, doing up to ten reps
* For lateral flex lower your left ear down toward your left shoulder and then your other ear to your right shoulder, up to ten reps
* For rotations just run your chin laterally toward your left should and then in the opposite direction, up to ten times

SHOULDER ROTATIONS

* Stand with shoulders back and knees slightly bent, shoulder width apart
* Bring left shoulder towards your left ear, bring it backwards, down and around and back to the starting point in a smooth and controlled action
* Do the same with the other side

ARM SWINGS

* Stand with feet shoulder width apart, knees slightly bent, back straight
* Overhead and back, swing each arm continuously up to overhead position and forward, down and then backwards, up to ten reps
* Side crossover, swing each arm to your side and cross affront your chest, up to ten reps

SIDE BENDING

* Stand tall, reach one arm up over head to the side and hold, repeat with other side, up to ten reps

TWISTS AND HIP CIRCLES

* For circles place hands on hips and feet a touch wider than shoulder width apart, make circles with your hips in one direction and then the other, repeat up to ten times
* For twists, arms at your sides, twist your hips and bottom to the left and back to the right, shifting your weight, repeat up to ten reps

MINI SQUAT

* Stand with feet shoulder width apart, back straight, head up and forward and hands in front
* Squat down until knees are parallel with floor
* Look straight ahead and think long
* Knees must point in the same direction as toes
* Straighten up and return to starting position
* Repeat up to ten reps

LEG SWINGS

* Flex and extend, stand beside wall sideways
* Place weight on right leg and have left hand on wall for balance
* Swing left leg in front and behind
* Do up to ten reps each side

DEEP LUNGE

* Stand upright with both feet together
* Lunge forward a full stride with left leg

* Left thigh should be parallel to ground
* Push back to starting position and repeat with other leg
* Up to ten reps each side

CALF STRETCH

* Facing wall place both hands on it and lung left leg back
will keeping right slightly bent and forward
* Raise and lower heel to feel calf stretch in back of leg
* Alternate each leg and repeat up to ten times each leg

These are some of the basic stretches to get you warmed up
for your workout each day. Make certain that you pay
attention to your body and concentrate on what you are
doing, don't just go through the motions.

And when you are training a specific body part hard make
certain to stretch it out thoroughly before and after each
session. This is going to ensure you get the maximum
benefits from your muscle building efforts and you are
going to remain injury-free. A must if you are going to get
big and fabulous in the muscle department!

The Split System
So what's the Split System? Well it's a system of weight
training that simply divides your training sessions by body
regions. Most likely you're familiar with upper and lower
body training.

Successful fitness trainers and bodybuilders tend to focus
on this system. And if you want to get even more focused
with this you will use numerous different combinations of
the main muscle group regions that are categorized for split
muscle training. Your main muscle group regions are:
* Chest
* Legs

- Butt
- Back
- Abs
- Arms

Most often people don't weight train in each of these specific regions, but rather combine them. Like arms, chest and back in one, and butt and legs in another. Of course ab training can be thrown in anywhere.

My advice is to experiment a little here. Figure out what works for you and develop a system. Depending on your specific goals you may be more or less focused in one area versus another. But keep in mind that you should NEVER neglect one area altogether because your body needs balance.

I'm sure you've seen those "chicken leg" bodybuilders at the gym. The ones that are "Hulksters" up top and have scrawny chicken legs below. UGH! Work with what you've got and aim for balance when all is said and done. Sound good to you?

Nutrition

Modern Fat Loss Techniques
Everybody and their dog want to believe there is a magic pill that zaps fat. Either that or some sort of mystic potion that only feeds off fat cells!

We want so much to believe this that we support and are a key contributor in the success of all fad diets. That's right! I think it's safe to say that every single person in the whole blinkin world has tried a "diet scheme" to try and drop weight faster than is physically possible. We've paid into it and used our ill formed thoughts to allow us believe that eating grapefruits for a week will make you drop ten pounds of fat and feel fabulous!

Or that cutting all carbs from your diet and just eating lean meats and lots of fresh juices will give you means to drop fifty pounds in just six weeks!

OMG! When will we ever learn? Guess we won't, but it's time for you to have a wake-up call. If you want to lose fat and build beautiful lean muscle you can. But you're going to have to work for it.

You will have to re-train yourself to choose healthy foods, exercise regularly and hold yourself to this. You will also need patience and reasonable expectations. Because if you don't the truth is YOU WILL FAIL!

Have a support system in place and most importantly a plan that is personalized to you! If you hate biking then don't do it for your cardio! You can do a bootcamp session, run or how about the cross-trainer? If you suck at getting up in the morning to workout then don't! Schedule your muscle building time for later in the day so that you know you have the best chances of sticking with it.

When it comes to eating, you are going to have to dig deep. Because how you fuel your body, when and how much, is a direct dictator of how successful you're going to be in your quest. If you eat crap, you'll feel like crap and you'll perform like crap.

With the help of a nutritionist you can learn what your body needs, all the essential vitamins and minerals it requires to perform for you. Giving you the energy you need to build muscle and get strong. Not to mention feeling fantastic about you!

So when it comes to the best route for losing weight, experts agree it's a combination of eating right and exercising regularly. By eating the right number of calories with the right foods, your body will be able to optimize energy and maximize results.

And by building muscle you are literally going to transform your body. Building muscles increases your metabolism simply because muscle burns more calories than fat does. It will leave you firmer and leaner. Basically you will be EYE-CANDY! Yummy!

Of course your food is important. To build muscle you need to eat the right amount of lean protein each day. Your body doesn't store or make protein so this is an absolute must. Good carbohydrates are required for long-lasting energy. So that you can push yourself to the extreme in your workouts and get results faster than last. And of course good fats are required to keep your systems running smoothly and to keep your psychosomatic on track.

Eating fat doesn't make your fat. Eating too much of the wrong kinds of fat will make you fat. If that makes sense!
With a combination of the right healthy eating and exercising you will lose fat and gain muscle. With hard work you can configure your body to do exactly what you want. And by making sure you expend more energy than you are ingesting you will progress consistently. By mixing it up and ensuring you have diversity in your eating and muscle building routine you will be WOWED at the results you get!

Carbohydrates and Fats

Here we're going to talk about carbs and fats. First we'll tackle carbohydrates from the very beginning.

So what are carbohydrates?

Good question! Technically they are starches and sugars that give energy to your body and its systems.

What's the difference between a "Good Carb" and a "Bad Carb??"

To simplify things we refer to carbohydrates as "good" and "bad." A bad carb is white bread, French fries, pastries and anything with nutrition less simple sugars. They break down quick, give you a fast shot of energy and then shoot you into low mode before you know it.

A good carb on the other hand is what your body needs. Whole grains and vegetables are good carbs; they take longer to breakdown, provide able nutrients and leave you energized longer than bad carbs do.

Good carbs are loaded with fiber and this means the nutrients in them are absorbed slowly into your system, helping to keep blood sugars level and your moods on par. I think you know what I'm getting at here.

So why do we need good carbohydrates?

Well carbohydrates lower your risk for chronic disease and it's recommended you get up to 65% of your calories from carbs, 20-30% from good fat and 10-35% from lean protein sources.

And the only way you can get fiber into your body is through plant sources. Did you know that? Fruits and vegetables are full of fiber. Fiber helps to decrease your risk for heart disease and also help prevent certain kinds of cancer and help control your weight.

Now let's look into fats. As you are likely aware there are good and bad fats too. Let's dive into GOOD FATS first.

First I'd like to gently remind you that to live you need fat. Fats are an integral part of being healthy. Some benefits of fat are:

- Providing essential fatty acids
- Keeping skin soft
- Fat-soluble vitamins
- Energy

And of course the problem in society today seems to be that we are getting way too much fat. Which of course causes all sorts of health issues that could be prevented.

Unsaturated fat or mono and poly-unsaturated fats are what you need in your diet. Some examples are:

- Corn Oil
- Fish Oil
- Canola Oil
- Almond Oil
- Soybean Oil
- Sunflower Oil
- Peanut Butter
- Nuts and Seeds

Good fats help with monitoring your nerve activity, help with vitamin absorption, immune system function and keeping your cells healthy. Omega-3 fats help reduce inflammation and boost your metabolism. So you can see there are huge benefits to including healthy fats in your diet.

Now let's have a look at the bad guys - BAD FATS

Bat fats are also knows as saturated fats and they will wreak havoc with your system. Clogging things up and accumulating within your body because it just doesn't know how to get rid of them. This of course triggers serious disease and of course obesity.

Some examples of these nasty fats are:

- Butter
- Lunch Meat
- Lard
- Animal Skin
- Full Fat Dairy Foods
- Partially Hydrogenated Oils
- Coconut Products

Bad fats seem to be hidden in the convenience foods we seem to crave. Fast foods, cakes and pastries, and pretty much every "junky" thing you can think of is loaded with bad fat!

Any food that's not natural, is processed and packaged is likely something you should stay clear of. I think you know what I'm getting at here!

Saturated fats will increase your LDL or bad cholesterol. Which of course isn't a good thing for you. And trans-fats were invented by scientist and they are basically liquid oils that stand up better in food production and help foods last longer on the shelf. French fries and even some microwave popcorn have unhealthy trans-fats within.

If you want to lose weight, build lean muscle and get ripped, you're going to have to cut out excess bad fats to start. This will help your body to unload all the accumulated toxins within and turn the corner to better health overall. How does this sound to you?

The Food Groups
Think WAY back to Primary school. Where you learned the basics about what foods you should and shouldn't eat. Not much of that has changed except maybe now we look at things in a little more detail. I'll start at the bottom and work my way up so you understand what you need to eat and why. You've gotta start somewhere right?

Every single move you make requires energy. And where do you get this energy from? Well food of course! In order for your car to run you need to feed it fuel, and in order for your mind and body to work you need to eat!

And what some people fail to recognize is that what you eat determines your physical composition, your mood and energy levels, and just how efficiently your body is going to run and process food as a whole.

Healthy eaters tend to be full of energy, they're leaner and more muscular, have better moods, and overall outlook on life. The opposite is true of couch potatoes that opt for fast-food venues and sweet treats.

Specifically there are 6 main food groups:

- Fruits
- Vegetables
- Grains
- Proteins Foods
- Dairy
- Oils

To simplify things I'm going to make them into 4 simple groups:

- Breads and Healthy Whole Grains
- Fruits and Vegetables
- Lean Meats and Alternates
- Low-Fat Dairy Products and Alternatives

We already know you need healthy unsaturated fats as well, and this can be accommodated nicely through just plain healthy eating! I don't think there are very many people in the world that have to worry about not getting enough fat in their diet!

IMPORTANT NOTE! Never forget that making sure your body is adequately hydrated is critical in life. Especially when you are weight training and exercising. Your body is composed mainly of water, and in order to keep all your systems functioning optimally you need to drink water.

The rule of thumb is 6-8 glasses a day, and on the days you are training you need to add at least 3-4 more. Drinking before, during and after exercising will ensure your body has the water stores it requires to stay energized and help you reach your goals.

Becoming dehydrated stresses your body and leaves you feeling lethargic and even ill. And did you know that by the time you "feel" thirsty you are already becoming dehydrated?

So by making a habit of quenching your thirst with water regularly you won't ever have to worry about short-changing yourself!

Oh, and water, herbal tea and clear soups should be your liquids of choice. Soda, coffee and other sports energy drinks and juices are not optimum here because they either instigate dehydration or are loaded with excess sugar and calories.

Okay - The Four Basic Food Groups Detailed

Breads and Healthy Whole Grains

Healthy Whole Grains are low in fat and high in fiber. This means they'll help you to feel full longer, purge toxins from your system and even reduce your risk of heart disease. Variety is key here and choosing from brown rice, oats, wild rice, quinoa, barley, oatmeal and whole wheat pasta are all fantastic for your mind and body.

There is a bit of a range here but experts agree that 4-6 servings here are adequate.

Fruits and Vegetables

This may be news to you but fruits and vegetables should be the largest food group for you each and every day. Fruits and vegetables are loaded with healthy antioxidants, which fight those nasty free-radicals trying to make you ill. They are also chalk full of all sorts of essential vitamins and minerals that are directly responsible for your great health.

Eating plenty of this food group everyday will also help to reduce your chances of developing various cancers and heart disease. Bright colors and textures are encouraged and making sure you eat fruits and vegetables with every meal and as snacks are going to do your body good.

8-10 servings of fruits and vegetables are what your body requires EACH day.

Being low in fat and calories and high in water content for the most part will also aid you in melting fat and building lean muscle. Steamed, baked, barbecued and stir-fried are preferred cooking methods and great choices include:

- Spinach
- Broccoli
- Romaine Lettuce
- Sweet Potatoes
- Carrots
- Bananas
- Blueberries/Blackberries/Raspberries/Strawberries
- Oranges
- Mangoes
- Kiwi
- Pears
- Pineapple
- Apples
- Papaya

And of course it's always beneficial to have a piece of fruit instead of a glass of juice.

Lean Meats and Alternatives

Meats and Alternatives will give your body important nutrients including protein, fat, zinc, magnesium, iron, B vitamins and magnesium. 2-3 serving per day is all you need. And at least two of these servings per week needs to come from fish sources; herring, char, trout, salmon and sardines.

Trimming fat before preparing is a smart move and baking, roasting, grilling, steaming and poaching are optimal cooking methods to keep fat low.

And did you know that all foods derived from meat, seafood, poultry, eggs, soy products, beans and peas, seeds and nuts, are part of this group?

Specific examples are:

- Pork
- Beef
- Chicken
- Lamb
- Veal
- Cashews
- Almonds
- Peanut Butter
- Eggs
- Sesame Seeds
- Pumpkin Seeds
- Sunflower Seeds
- Tuna
- Cod
- Trout
- Salmon
- Snapper
- Halibut

- Herring
- Catfish
- Shellfish
- Beans
- Chickpeas
- Soy Products

It's very important here to choose low-fat varieties because the extra fat added in preparation and in meat choices can make them unhealthy. For instance, you can have a healthy portion of low-fat chicken. But if you choose fattier thighs and deep fry them in a hydrogenated rich batter, you are transforming this meat serving into something very unhealthy. Do you understand what I'm saying?

Be smart in your meat servings and you'll build your muscles and mind strong!

Low-Fat Dairy Products and Alternatives

Your body needs dairy products and alternatives to keep your bones healthy and strong; also reducing your risk of osteoporosis. This will also reduce your risk of dealing with heart disease and type 2 diabetes. Along with lowering your blood pressure, regulating bodily systems, and helping your skin and structure to remain vibrant and healthy.

Many milk products are fortified with Vitamin D to help maintain adequate levels of phosphorous and calcium.

Some common dairy products to eat are:

- Skim Milk
- Low Fat Milk
- Low Fat Cheese

- Ice-Cream
- Yogurt
- Soy Milk
- Almond Milk

Calcium is very important in ensuring your body remains healthy and strong for the long run. If you skimp here your body will naturally break down and your skeletal structure for one will pay the price. In severe situations your bones can actually get soft and bend. One serious result that is a symptom and reality of osteoporosis.

Okay, now that you've got the basics we're going to venture in a little further

Food and Weight Training

To each his/her own right? Well this book is geared towards Modern Bodybuilding Techniques, and I also know that you will have different goals here than "Bob" or "Maddy" might. Regardless of these differences, there will be times where you take a directional shift in your training and nutrition plan.

Some may weight train to build big hunky muscles while others may want to drop weight and tone their body. Both in which muscles benefit. Bottom line is your diet and nutrition plan have a huge voice in whether or not your hit your goals or fall off the beaten path yet again.

You will learn very quickly that different nutrients in varying amounts are needed for your specific goal. If you'd like to bulk up by building your muscle mass then you'll need to consume plenty of lean protein. On the flip side if you are trying to lean up and get shredded before a competition you'll need less in the calorie department overall.

Another interesting fact before we continue is that you can't ever change the number of fat or muscle cells your body has. What you were born with is what you've got to work with. But what you can do is shrink or grow them. And of course this is dependent on your lifestyle, exercise and eating habits, genetics, attitude, and health status. Some of which is controllable and some which isn't.

Now let's move forward and talk about Vitamins and Minerals as they are critical in your overall good health and muscle building goals.

Vitamins and Minerals
For one vitamins don't have usable energy when your body breaks them down. What they do is help enzymes that release energy from fats, carbs and protein. Suffice to say, minerals and vitamins are readily available in the natural foods we eat. So relax before you reach for your gummy multivitamin!

Here are a few of the key vitamins you need and their functions. This will help you understand better why you need certain foods to build your muscles and body strong.

Thiamin - It helps with metabolism and specific nerve function and can be found in foods like watermelon, spinach, green peas, lean ham and pork and soy milk.

Riboflavin (B2) - Assists in metabolism, sight and your beautiful skin. Broccoli, spinach, milk and eggs are awesome sources.

Niacin (B3) - Also helps with metabolism, your skin healthy, nervous and digestive system. Foods to provide niacin are potatoes, spinach, lean beef, tuna and chicken breast.

Biotin - Helps with fat synthesis, amino acid metabolism, and glycogen synthesis and energy metabolism. It's found in lots of different foods.

Pantothenic Acid - Is key in supporting energy metabolism and is also found in many different foods.

Pyridoxine (B6) - Helps with fatty acid and amino acid metabolism and red blood cell production. You can find this vitamin in chicken breast, bananas, broccoli, squash, spinach and potatoes.

Folate - Assists with formation of new cells and DNA synthesis. This is especially important in the proper development of a baby. Foods that are good sources are asparagus, spinach, broccoli, tomato juice, green beans, lentils and beans.

B12 - Is used for new cell creation, breaking down amino acids and fatty acids and supporting nerve cell function. It's commonly found in milk, eggs, fish, chicken and meats.

Ascorbic Acid - Used for the metabolism of amino acids, synthesis of collagen, immunity, iron absorption and reproduction. This vitamin is found in kiwi, mango, oranges, strawberries, broccoli spinach, red pepper and tomato juice.

Retinol (A) - Helps with vision, teeth and bone health, skin, reproduction and to strengthen the immune system.

Foods like mango, tomato juice, sweet potatoes, broccoli, carrots and butternut squash are superb sources.

D - Helps with bone mineralization. And you can get it with pure sunshine, egg yolk, fatty fish and fortified milk.

E - This is an antioxidant. It regulates oxidation reactions and assists with cell membrane stabilization. You can find it in soybean, corn and canola oils, wheat germ, tofu, avocado, sunflower seeds, tofu and sweet potato.

K - Helps with blood-clotting protein formation and regulates the calcium in your blood. Foods that are great sources are spinach, Brussels sprouts, cabbage and leafy green vegetables.

Now let's take a gander at some important minerals your body needs to keep your mind and body smiling.

Sodium - Helps with electrolyte and fluid balance, contributes to your muscles contracting and nerve impulses. Meats, milk, soy sauce, bread and of course salt are decent choices.

Chloride - Assists in keeping fluids and electrolytes level and helps process food.

Potassium - Also helps balance electrolytes and fluids, cell strength, nerve function and muscle contraction. Foods that are great here are broccoli, squash, carrots, avocado, bananas, strawberries, milk and cod.

Calcium - Helps with teeth and bone health and assists with blood clotting. Cheese, yogurt, tofu, broccoli, spinach and green beans are great sources.

Phosphorus - Assists in forming cells, teeth and bones and also contributes to acid-base balance. All animal foods are great sources.

Magnesium - Is partial to supporting bone mineralization, muscle contraction, protein building, immunity and nerve transmission. Foods that are great sources are sunflower seeds, cashews, halibut, broccoli, spinach, tomatoes and navy beans.

Iron - Helps with hemoglobin and carrying oxygen throughout your body. Great sources are tofu, green beans, broccoli, spinach, parsley, artichoke and shrimp.

Zinc - Found in many enzymes and in making proteins. It helps transport vitamin A, in healing, sperm formation, and fetal development and in tasting. Excellent sources are broccoli, spinach, lentils, green peas, turkey, lean ground beef, lean steak, Swiss cheese and plain yogurt.

Selenium - An antioxidant that helps shield the body from oxidation with the help of vitamin E. Whole grains, meats and seafood are fabulous sources.

Iodine - Helps to regulate metabolism, development and growth. It's found in cheese, milk, whole grain bread, salt and seafood.

Copper - It's required for the absorption and use of iron. It also helps form hemoglobin and various enzymes. Meats and water are good sources.

Manganese - Assists with many different cells functions and is found in lots of different foods.

Fluoride - Is critical in the formation of teeth and bones and helps to deter cavities from setting in. Tea, seafood and water with fluoride are good sources.

Chromium - Closely linked with insulin and is necessary to release energy from glucose. You can find this mineral in nuts, cheese, grains, yeast and vegetable oils.

Molybdenum - Interlinked with various cell processes. Organ meats and legumes have this mineral.

So you can see you've got to eat a whole lot of healthy foods to get all the vitamins and minerals your body needs to fight off free radicals and stay disease free. And to give you the energy and ability to build muscle, burn fat and get strong.

And many people will opt for supplementation to be certain they give their body everything it requires to serve them well. That's all fine and dandy, but remember that natural food sources are the best way to get them. Why? Well because they are readily absorbed by a healthy body and more enjoyable!

Synthetic vitamins and minerals not taken in the right combination may shoot right through your system. It's a tough call. So food sources first with supplement backup should serve you well!

And when you are weight training it's even more important that you make certain you are getting all your vitamins and minerals. Eating healthy foods in the right amounts regularly will give you everything you need to make your muscle dreams come true.

Gaining Weight

Many people looking to Bodybuild want to gain weight. And when you do this you can opt to do it in the form of fat, muscle and/or water. Serious Bodybuilders will bulk up with some extra fat on the off-season so they can start seriously training again and transform this extra fat into bigger muscles!

Water weight comes and goes depending on what you are eating, your training goals and your hormones.

In theory if you want to gain weight you need to consume more calories that you expend. So you need to eat more and decrease your activity level.

However most people who want to gain weight for weight training purposes or just to fill out their scrawny frame a little, they want to gain muscle. Makes sense right?

Gaining muscle also means you are putting your scale number up with health in mind and that's all good. Your body prefers muscle on it compared to fat, but also keep in mind your body does need fat to function properly. Did you know that if you don't have enough fat on your body your brain will actually start to take on a mind of its own?

Scary stuff!

Never mind that stuff for now though because too little fat is most often the least of our worries!

So let's have a look at someone wanting to build bulk. Maybe you're tired of being the spaghetti string guy on the block and what to become a solid mass of walking muscle - or something like that anyway.

Here are a few key factors that will help you do just that! Gain muscle and get that body you have always dreamed off to strut your stuff.

* Maximize your Muscle Building

If you want to gain muscle you're going to have to up your protein intake. Your body has very short-term reserves of protein called protein synthesis. But they are always being utilized with the rest of your bodily processes requiring protein. Manufacturing hormones, for example.

This means there's less protein readily available in your body to make muscles.

So what's the simple solution?

Just eat more! What you need to actually do is build and temporarily store proteins faster than your body is breaking down the ones you have. Do this and you will have the platform and ability to begin gaining muscle.

* Munch Away on Meat

Technically what you want to do is aim for at least 1 gram of protein per pound that you weight. Or in the metric system you should be around 2.2 grams per 1Kg's of bodyweight. Essentially this is the maximum amount your body is able to use per day. So if you weigh 180 pounds (81Kg's), then you need 180 grams of protein per day.

So yes you are going to have to start paying attention to how much protein is in the food you eat, and make the adjustments to make it happen. Yes it can be a tad overwhelming at first, but it won't take you long to get used to it.

And just to give you a ballpark menu of what this "Joe" would have to eat to get his 180 grams of protein, here's an example.

- An 8oz (226 grams) chicken breast
- 1 1/2 cups cottage cheese
- A roast beef sandwich
- Three eggs
- A full glass of milk
- 3 ounces of cashews

* Consume More Calories

So you need more protein, but you will also need more calories overall. Experts agree there are about 3500 calories (14.65 KJs) in a pound. So technically in order to gain one pound, you need to eat 3500 calories (1 Kg= 37,000KJs) more than your body uses each day.

This is factoring in your regular exercise and normal eating routine and lifestyle. So let's say you need to eat 3000 calories each day right now to keep your weight constant. This means you will have to add at least another 3500 calories each week in order to gain one single pound. Now don't forget to take your training into consideration here too. If you are burning more calories lifting weights than you normally do, it's important that you add extra energy to your body to compensate for that. Remember you want to stay ahead of the game and bulk your body up, not slim it down!

* Focus on your Biggest Muscles

Now if you are just starting to get into the exercise routine it really won't take much to urge your body into protein synthesis mode. But if you've been training for a while you are better to focus directly on your big muscles to get bulky fast.

Your big muscle groups are your back, chest, legs to start. So making sure your routine has lots of squats, bench presses, pull ups, dead lifts, military presses and bent-over rows is going to help you get bulky big fast!

Make sure you are lifting heavier weights, so you're doing less reps and allotted less rest time in between sets.

* Drink Up Before Lifting

Of course drinking and driving is a "no-no" but there's no law against drinking and lifting! Studies show that people who drink an amino acid and carbohydrate filled shake before working out gained more muscle than those who didn't.

This makes sense because you're giving your body exactly what it needs to trigger protein synthesis. And take note that because exercising gets your juices flowing, this might very well help you absorb and utilize all those yummy carbs and amino acids you just ingested - and faster.

Also take note you'll need up to 20 grams of protein with each shake. This is basically a scoop of whey-protein powder.

And if you aren't a shake drinker don't fret because there is another way. You can also do it with old-fashioned eating! A chicken breast sandwich with real cheese on whole wheat bread will also do the same trick. Although this will take a little longer to get into your system. So take that into consideration when you're in planning mode.

* Lift on Alternate Days

If you want to gain weight and build muscle you can't overdo it. So many people get excited and try to burn up the gym every day and this just doesn't work. You'll fatigue your body and mind and this is only going to break you down. Stressing your system and actually encouraging your body to break down your muscles to use as energy because you will be taxing your system too much.

Studies show that a good workout will increase your protein synthesis for a good 48 hours after. Remembering your muscles will grow while you're RESTING. So it's very important you use this fact to your advantage, and make certain that you make the best decisions for you to bulk up fast!

* Carb Up After

It's not just about working out and forgetting. If you want to gain weight and build muscle you are going to need to give your body good carbs. What happens is that meals with carbs after your workout will help to increase your insulin levels. And this will literally slow down the rate in which your body breaks down proteins.

It's not a huge deal but make certain you have good carbs close at hand after you've exhausted yourself. Grab a peanut butter sandwich on whole grain bread or a banana and all will be well!

* Fuel Your Body Every 2-3 Hours

Yes this may seem like a lot but it really isn't. I'm not asking you to sit down and have a buffet every few hours.

What I'm suggesting is that you eat a little something every couple of hours in order to communicate to your body through action that you want it to increase the length of protein synthesis. Your body doesn't understand words so you have to "show" it what you want it to do.

So just figure out how many calories you need to eat each day and divide it by 6 or 7. And of course remember to get at least 20 grams of protein with each mini-meal. It may take a little time but eventually your mind and body will connect and you'll see it in your weight!

* Indulge in Ice-Cream Once a Day

Now don't go all crazy on me here. Funny how experts have found that having a bowl of ice-cream after your workout will trigger your insulin levels to rise the fastest! Keeping in mind there is too much of a good thing. And did you know this will also help to deter your body from naturally breaking down protein after training?

* There's Truth to Warm Milk Before Bed

I don't know about you but my grandmother always used to tell me a warm glass of milk before bed would help me sleep better. I don't know about that, but I do know that combined snacks of good carbs and protein are incredibly important when gaining weight through healthy muscle building.

Funny thing is that when you sleep milk is more likely to stick with you and deter protein breakdown from happening. Maybe you want a cup of raisin bran with skim milk, or a cup of cottage cheese with some fruit. And don't forget to eat again right after you wake up.

If you stick to this plan you are going to get results a whole lot faster than you would otherwise. Believe it!

In Addition

Many people that are trying to gain weight through weight training think that all sports beverages are created equal and they're not. More sports drinks are LOADED with sugars and this is going to upset your stomach and give you bowel issues that you don't want me to get into.

Bottom line is by drinking sports beverages before and during workouts you're just literally flushing your money straight down the toilet.

And if you are going to use a shake before your workout make sure it's a whey protein one. This is going to give your body the punch it needs to maximize your workout and give your body the ability to build muscle instead of breaking it down.

Does this make sense?

Weight Loss
On the flip side here are people that want to lose weight. This doesn't mean you don't want to build beautiful lean muscle but maybe you have a few rolls you'd like to take out the curb too. No worries. Building muscle and losing weight is the most effective and efficient way to lose weight and keep it off.

This is what your body has been programmed to do. It's just that we've short-circuited everything throughout our lives, and caused huge disconnect between our physical and our mental.

So yes you can go on another FAD Diet and drop a few pounds fast. Most of it is water weight that you're going to gain back depressingly fast at some point.

Or you can go crazy with the workouts and not bother changing your eating much. This will give you some weight loss initially but soon you will get tired of overexerting yourself and when you do your scale numbers will rocket straight up.

Experts agree the best route to lose weight and sustain your loss is to get a new brain! Well technically that's not exactly right but it is the idea. What I mean is that you are going to need to re-train your brain by learning new healthy habits. Because obviously you're not satisfied with what you're doing right now - right?

So by making better food choices and getting your butt into the gym to build lean muscle, you are going to get a smoking hot body while sending your fat packing. The hard route my friends is one or the other. Combine the two and you will reach your goals a heck of a lot faster and with permanence. Besides, aren't you tired of losing the same twenty pounds every year?

Now if you are into professional body building you'll be well aware of the "bulking" and "cutting" phases. Body builders are extremists and when they gain weight they do it with attitude. When they need to lean out they pull every punch to drop fat and water weight FAST. And we're not going to get into whether or not this is healthy because that's a whole other book!

If you want to lose fat or weight and build some muscle you need to do three things:

- Eat Healthy
- Lift Weights
- Do Cardio

The focus here needs to shift a little and to ensure you are doing regular intense cardiovascular activity at least 5 days a week. What this does is naturally trigger your fat burning mode, and this means you are programming your body to always be using energy. Think of this as a "base" move towards your ultimate goal of fat loss.

You also need to eat regularly and in the right amounts to support his shift of motive. You need to let your body know you are going to feed it regularly and enough, but you aren't going to give it so much that it's going to want to store any of it. This is an intricate balance that you may need a professional to help you find.

You're also going to need to stick with the weight training in order to build your muscles. You just don't necessarily have to lift so heavy and you don't need to take in as many calories each day to support this. You don't want to short yourself on the fuel but you also don't want to overdo it or your body will have a tough time burning your fat stores.

Are you following all of this?

Weight Loss = Less Energy In + More Energy Out

And you can do this with all sorts of different combinations.

Maintenance
We've touched on this here and there. And where people seem to "fail" is in the maintenance department. People hit their goal of losing weight by creating new healthy habits

only to fall back into their unhealthy comfort zone which of course brings with it weight gain.

We are creatures of habit and it takes a heck of a lot of accountability and dedication to lose weight and keep it off for good. This involves a lifestyle change that is thought of as permanent. You need to actually change your daily eating and workout patterns in order to hit your weight loss goals and keep them.

Because if you hit your goals and then don't bother holding yourself accountable to the new behavior, you will fall straight backwards and have to climb that hill all over again.

You know you and have to figure out the best route for you to stay on track for life. Learn how to manage a few slips and slides and still stick with your guns. I will suggest however, a few strategies that should assist you in your quest of healthy change. Read through them and use the ones that will benefit you best. Be strong and determined, and DO NOT let yourself make excuses of any sort.

Excuses will be your avenue to failure - TRUST ME!

* Become a Planner

What happens with many people is that something unexpected arises, and they don't know how to deal with it. They haven't planned and aren't expecting it, and allow their mental to make the best of this surprise. Often minor derailments are the trigger for ultimate weight gain.

This is especially important when it comes to your eating and drinking. Set yourself up for success my friend. Mentally prepare yourself and you'll do fine. To start having regular snacks or mini-meals throughout the day is a great way to manage your hunger, keep your blood sugars and moods level, and avoid any "starvation" moments. You know the ones that trigger major pig-out sessions! A few other pointers here are:

- No sampling while cooking.
- If you're hungry between meals drink a glass of water first.
- If you want to snack switch your focus to a physical activity fast.
- Make dinner the last thing you eat before breakfast.
- Measure everything to start. Especially when snacking or you'll eat the whole box.

* Easy on the Booze

In case you didn't know alcohol punches a wallop of calories with basically no nutrients. Of course the number of calories varies and a lite beer is a much better choice than a fancy mixed drink. A Margarita can run you up to 600 calories - For One!

A glass of wine is okay at around 100 calories and a hard liquor drink with diet pop runs you just under a hundred calories. The idea here is to limit your alcohol to a glass or two occasionally.

Make smart choices here and you'll be able to relax and have a little fun without having to deal with the double baggage. A hangover and some extra fat just for fun.

* Keep Meals Positive

Try to make your eating times about more than eating food. Make it a positive social event you enjoy with friends and family.

- Eat slowly
- Chew your food
- Don't watch television or play on your cell phone while eating

* Use Meals to Help You Control Your Intake

You need to learn to:

Plan Meals
- Eat When You're Hungry
- Limit How Much You Eat Out

* Get Your Heart Rate Up

Now I can think of lots of different ways to do this but let's just stick with regular exercise for now.

If you get at least 5 hours of exercise in every week studies have shown you have a better shot at losing weight and keeping it off. This makes sense because your mind and body are going to recognize the benefits of training. And this is key in helping people to stick with it.

* Accountability

It is very important for you to make sure you have accountability factors in place. Whether you are stepping on the scale a few times a week, checking in with a trainer or having a friend keep tabs on you, it's all important in sustainability.

We need to "see" things in order to believe them and we need to do it again and again and again in order to turn it into habit. Help yourself by holding yourself accountable for your weight loss and your actions. This is only going help you psychosomatically and physically. And that sexy swimsuit or trim and hunky swim trunks are going to fit your year after year!

Motivation

In General we need motivation to do just about everything in life. From getting out of bed in the morning, to getting our butt to the gym. Money may be your motivator to get out of bed and get to work because if you don't show up you don't get paid.

Maybe an upcoming family reunion is a motivating factor to get you to lose weight. Perhaps an old school friend has inspired or motivated you to build muscle because he just competed in his first body building competition and won.

We need motivators to "make" us do things.

Maybe you just lost a close family member and this motivated you to start looking for a serious relationship so you won't end up alone like they were. Or perhaps you visited an old-age home and that motivated you to sell your house and travel the world. To experience life to the fullest before you end up with no choice but to sit in a chair and watch it pass you by.

Motivation is fantastic if we use it positively.

Motivation to Exercise

So why is it so hard for people to get motivated to exercise? We know we "should" be exercising, but we just toss out excuse after excuse to make sure it just doesn't happen.

Why? Why? Why?

Fact is change is tough to say the least. Good or bad, healthy or unhealthy, we are conditioned to stay as we are, and it takes a heck of a lot of effort to make any sort of change in our life. That's what makes it so tough to lose weight!

To get yourself headed in the right direction here are a few pointers.

* Make it Personal

You need to figure out what's important to you and find a personal reason to get your butt off the couch and get exercising. Maybe it's as simple as getting weighed at the doctors and being ticked at the number.

You know there are oodles of benefits to getting fit and healthy. Figure out which ones are important to you and use them. Even just going for a walk every morning will help you to:

- Think clearer and be positive
- Kick-start your metabolism and get to burning fat
- Keep you from overeating at breakfast and throughout the day
- Lower your risk of developing all sorts of serious health conditions
- Show your children that you care about your health

Perhaps your motivation could be as simple as the positive social experience you get from a yoga class. Meeting your friends for some fun and invigorating exercise could very well be something you look forward to for a long time to come.

* Set Yourself Up For Success

Make sure you set reasonable expectations for yourself to get fit and healthy. If you jump out of the starting gates expecting to run a marathon three weeks after starting, you're just setting yourself up to fail!

My advice is to sit down with a trainer and make a plan. One with specific goals that you know you're going to hit, especially to start. This will at least enable you to know that you can lose weight and get healthy and keep it that way.

Start slow and work your way up. If you go too crazy with changes too fast you may get overwhelmed at scoot back into your old and unhealthy ways. We all know what that's about I think.

* Change Your Mentality

Stop focusing on exercise as exercise, if that makes sense? Figure out what sort of physical activity you enjoy and stick with it. You can have fun and lose weight. If you hate enclosed spaces with lots of people then don't train in the gym during busy times.

Maybe go in when it's not so busy or perhaps take up swimming or biking to begin. It really doesn't matter what you do, but you are setting yourself up to win if you make it fun.

Another very important point to always remember is NEVER QUIT. You need to understand this road to building your body big and strong is full of the unexpected. Ups and downs are going to happen and you need to be mentally prepared not to let them deter you from your goals.

Allow for "pauses" in your plans and be forgiving of yourself. One pig-out day can't ruin everything, or sleeping through your alarm on a training day doesn't make you bad. What's important is what you do afterwards. By picking yourself up and refocusing on your set goals, you will eventually be kind to yourself and allow for a little bend here and there without breaking yourself in two.

Never quit and you can only win in the long run and it's the long run that counts my friend. BELIEVE IT!

Now that you're armed and dangerous and I think it's time for you to get building! I think it's time for you to apply your DACT Method to your Modern Bodybuilding Techniques!

References

Chapman, D. (2012). Eugen Sandow: Bodybuilding's Great Pioneer. from http://www.eugensandow.com/

Gerard Tortora, N. A. (1984). *Principles of Anatomy and Physiology* (fourth ed.). New Your: Harper & Row.

Gwillim, S. (2012). All About Bodybuilding Techniques [Electronic Version]. *CriticalBench.com.* Retrieved 16/11/12 from http://www.criticalbench.com/bodybuilding_technique.htm.

Howells, M. (2012). How Does Classic Bodybuilding Differ From Modern Bodybuilding? [Electronic Version]. Retrieved 15-11-12 from http://www.wisegeek.com/how-does-classic-bodybuilding-differ-from-modern-bodybuilding.htm.

Hoxha, T. (1995). How Joe and Ben Weider Became the Founding Fathers of Bodybuilding. September 1995 issue. Retrieved 18/11, 2012, from http://www.getbig.com/articles/faq-wdr.htm

Jim Manion, C. I. P. L. (2007-09-26). Chairman IFBB Professional League. In I. P. League (Ed.).

Littman, J. (2012). Bodybuilding And The Olympics: An Ongoing Controversy. Retrieved 2008-08-19

Wikipedia. (2012a). Bodybuilding. Retrieved 18/11, 2012, from http://en.wikipedia.org/wiki/Bodybuilding

Wikipedia. (2012b). Joe Weider. Retrieved 18/11, 2012, from http://en.wikipedia.org/wiki/Joe_Weider

Images courtesy of patrisyu at FreeDigitalPhotos.net http://www.freedigitalphotos.net/images/acknowledgement.php

1   -----ego te provoco-----

www.ingramcontent.com/pod-product-compliance
Lightning Source LLC
Chambersburg PA
CBHW070551290526
45790CB00002B/638